Paleo Diet
for Beginners
Volume 1

By Anas Malla

Table of Contents

Introduction

I want to thank you and congratulate you for purchasing the book "**Paleo Diet for Beginners!**"

This book contains proven steps and strategies on how to lose weight with the Paleo diet, as well as all the required information on how to live the healthy Paleo lifestyle.

Do you think you have overweight or obesity issues? Do you believe that the way you eat negatively affects your health? Would you like to find out a way to live a healthy lifestyle that will benefit you in long-term?

If the answer to the questions mentioned above is yes, then Paleo diet is the right choice for you. It will help you reach your ideal weight, but more importantly, it will help you maintain it! Furthermore, it will lead to you feeling much better and being more energized.

Let's take a look at the areas we will cover in the book:

- **Paleo diet overview** – what is Paleo nutrition and how it works; all essential information you need to know
- **Complete food guide on Paleo diet** – we give you an in-depth look at foods you should eat and those you should avoid when living the Paleo lifestyle. You also get a guide for eating out, and we discuss whether you need nutritional supplements

- **Benefits of the Paleo diet** – how exactly will it help you; we list a whole bunch of ways it positively influences your health
- **How to start the Paleo diet**? - The toughest thing to do when making a transition to the new way of nutrition is to start. Fortunately, we have some essential tips for you

And much more!!

Everything you need to know about the Paleo diet is in one place – here.

Thanks again for purchasing this book, I hope you enjoy it!

Paleo Diet Overview

What Is Paleo Diet?

At the very beginning, let's try to give a short explanation on what Paleo nutrition is. If I had to describe it in a single sentence, I would say that it is a diet that switches the modern approach to food with an ancient one and offers to secure optimal health by eating whole and unprocessed foods.

Yes, you heard it right; Paleo diet focuses on the ways our ancestors from thousands of years ago consumed their meals. Paleo is short for Paleolithic, which marks the early phase of the Stone Age. Paleo diet means that you should eat like your caveman ancestors!

They used two methods for finding their food. The first one is hunting, a way they used to secure meat and fish for themselves. The other technique is gathering, and it was a way of securing vegetables, fruits, nuts, and seeds. That means that there is no room for cereals, pasta, or sweets in your nutrition. In fact, you can't eat anything that people couldn't hunt or gather in caveman times.

Fortunately, our ancestors also didn't have a way to track the amount of calories they consume. That means that the Paleo way of nutrition doesn't require you to count calories each day. Instead, you only need to focus on eating the right foods. So, if you hate all those diets that are obsessing about how many grams of a particular food you can eat, relax, Paleolithic diet won't ask this from you.

Even without counting calories, Paleo diet will secure that you reach your ideal weight and shed those extra pounds. However, the most significant advantage is that it will ensure the optimal health of your body and improve the overall state of your organism. We will focus on the benefits of the Paleo way of nutrition later. For now, let's say that it is in your interest to do everything right. You should focus on proper foods and adjust your mindset to eating like a caveman. If you manage to do this, Paleo nutrition might just be the best thing that ever happened to you.

Our genetics hadn't changed much since our ancestors hunted and gathered food. Unlike that, our way of nutrition significantly adjusted over the last century, and we implemented some rather unhealthy choices, including grains, cereals, and candy. The aim of the Paleo diet is to help you achieve the optimal state of your organism both regarding your weight and its health. It's a way of nutrition that can be used for the rest of your life. Unlike other diets that you can use only for a certain amount of time, Paleolithic lifestyle is there to stay and help you maintain your vitality and health.

You might have seen some pictures where our ancestors are portrayed. If you did, you could probably remember that each of those illustrations showed them in the same way – they were muscular, athletic, and they possessed incredible agility.

Now, let's compare that to how an average human looks today. I'm sure that you often feel sleep deprived, unhappy or stressed out. Do you have problems with your weight or maybe some chronic disease is haunting you? There is a good chance that your lifestyle is the cause of all this.

As you can see, there is a noticeable difference between how our ancestors looked like and how we look like. But what is the cause behind this change?

Believe it or not, it's agriculture. When homo sapiens discovered farming thousands of years ago, we quickly evolved from hunting and gathering to growing our food. That enabled us to settle down, and form societies and the evolution got quicker from that point. While that's obviously great because of all the technological quirks (one of them being the reason why you are reading this book), it also damaged our bodies by disrupting our nutrition.

Although it might seem that we had time to adjust to the new principle of nutrition, the human genome changed less than 0.02% in the last 40,000 years. A couple of thousands of years wasn't near enough to adjust our bodies to the increased amount of sugar and grains that we have been consuming lately.

There is a good metaphor used by Robb Wolf, a Paleo guru. Just think of a large football field that has the length of 100 yards. Now, we have been running 99 yards while hunting and gathering for food and our bodies got used to that system. Our diet has changed in the last yard, but our body cannot accustom to those changes.

According to the statistics, 66% of people in the United States consider themselves overweight, while every third person falls into the obese category. Something is wrong, and we have to react. The change that we need comes in the form of the paleo diet.

How it Works

It's quite simple – Paleolithic way of nutrition means that you should focus on eating meat, fish, veggies and seasonal fruits. It's just the way our ancestors did, and it's the only way to eat in a way that perfectly suits your organism. The Paleo diet focuses on eating in a way that our bodies were biologically designed to eat. That way we can use our genetic potential and become healthier in a matter of days.

Let's take a brief look at what happens when we go too far in consuming grains on a regular basis. Our organisms take the carbs from the grains and transform it into sugar. Our body can use that sugar in one of the following two ways – it can burn it as energy or store it as fat. You've heard it right; grains are probably what's causing you to be overweight, which is why the Paleo diet recommends quitting eating them.

If that does not reason enough for you to give up grains, let's also mention the damage that can be caused by gluten and lectins. There's been a lot of talk about gluten lately (I think the famous tennis player

Novak Djokovic spread it on a global basis) and there is reliable science behind that. You see, it turns out that most of the population is intolerant to gluten, although it is a protein. That is why the food producers are trying to offer gluten-free items. But have you asked about why most of the people on all sides of the world are gluten-intolerant? It's because their bodies weren't biologically designed to process gluten. Furthermore, consuming it regularly may lead to joint pain, dermatitis, acid reflux, and other health issues.

As for lectins, they are an ingredient you can find in grains that don't like our gastrointestinal tract. In fact, it prevents it from repairing itself, which can lead to considerable damage. Consider lectin as a natural toxin you can find in grains. That would mean that even grains evolved to contain ingredients that should make us avoid them!

Aside from grains, you should avoid sugar (unless the fruit is the source). Sugar leads to your blood sugar levels changing too rapidly, and that can cause a real chaos in our organisms. Now, let's sublime this section into a short sentence:

You should avoid grains, sugar, and processed foods. On the other hand, you should consume meat, fish, vegetables, seasonal fruits, nuts, and seeds.

This book offers you a complete food guide for being on Paleo diet where we will go into details for particular types of food you should eat and avoid.

However, the core of this way of nutrition is in the bolded sentence located above. If you do that, your overall well-being and your health will have both short-term and long-term benefits.

The Question of Energy

The Paleo diet recommends keeping your intake of carbohydrates at a low level. You might wonder, and you would have the right to do that, where do you get your energy from then?

Let's return once again to the biological design of the human body. Consuming fewer carbs hasn't been an issue for our ancestors, which means our organism is programmed to adapt to the lower amount of carbohydrates. In that case, our body starts using fat (the one we consume AND the one stored in our organism) for energy. That is the way how you will get rid of those extra pounds when you start the Paleo diet.

It's a win-win situation. Not only fewer carbs will cause less spikes of sugar in your organism, but it will start using fat as energy, which will lead to a decrease in fat storage and therefore reduce your fat percentage. That way you will look better than ever!

How Much Should You Eat?

As mentioned, you don't need to count your calories. In fact, you don't even have to look at the clock to see whether it's time for a meal. You are free to eat whenever you want (but make sure that you feel hungry). After all, cavemen didn't eat on schedule. Furthermore, they would sometimes go a day or more without any food. They managed to survive thanks to the fact that they turned their body into fat burning machines and used the excess fat when they are forced not to eat for days.

So, eat when you feel hungry. Don't feel the obligation to eat every couple of hours. In fact, you should focus on having full meals once you do decide to eat. There is no need to worry even if you skip a meal, just make sure that you don't eat a whole pizza and two burgers just because you feel hungry afterward.

You should only ensure that you find a good source of protein, such as eggs or chicken, to go with some vegetables and you've got yourself a meal. You can also consume seasonal fruits. If you feel like you are constantly hungry, you can also think about including some healthy fats, such as olive oil, avocado, almond butter, walnuts, almonds, etc.

The Importance of Fat

Fat has been victimized in public for the last several decades, and it now has a bad reputation. However, all those tips to reduce the intake of fat and increase carbs have gotten us...nowhere. Instead, we are fatter than ever before.

There is something you need to distinguish here; there are unhealthy fats, and there are HEALTHY fats. As long as you concentrate on consuming the latter ones, you can tap into your genetic potential and turn your body into a healthy fat-burning machine. We mentioned some of the healthy fats in this section, and we will tell you more about them in the food guide later.

The important thing to remember is that fat is not your enemy. In fact, in Paleo diet, it takes up a significant portion of nutrition. Our ancestors greatly benefitted from eating, and there is no reason why you can't.

The History behind the Paleo Diet

Now that we know what Paleo diet is and some of its basic mechanisms, it might be fun to take a look at the history of this diet and just how it came to be so popular. To trace how the Paleolithic diet originated, we need to go back about forty thousand years ago. That is approximately when our ancestors started hunting and gathering in order to survive. They were looking for animals and hunting them down in the woods, as well as gathering vegetables, fruits, and even nuts. So, if you are looking for a particular founder of the Paleo diet, that was nobody else but our ancestors.

Let's journey back to the early 1900s and get to meet Joseph Knowles, a man who spent two months in the wilderness of Maine. It was a miracle that he survived, but that was an adventure he was willing to take to prove his point.

What did Knowles do? He made a record of his vitals before going into the wilderness. During the time spent in the wild, he started surviving by eating berries. Not long has passed and he included meat and fish into his nutrition because he learned to hunt. He made shoes and clothes from tree bark. As you can see, it was a complete adventure with the goal of surviving.

When two months have passed, Knowles returned and visited the doctor. According to the available data, his health was in a better state than before. Eating like ancestors (hunting and gathering food) made his healthier and stronger.

However, there was no internet or other reliable channels to distribute this fantastic news at the time. That's why Paleo diet had to wait until the 1970s to become famous. That is when a gastroenterologist Walter L. Voegtlin started advocating that this particular diet can improve our overall well-being. He concluded this after realizing that Paleo nutrition helped his patients that had indigestion issues and IBS. He was the author of The Stone Age Diet: Based on In-depth Studies of Human Ecology and the Diet of Man, which was published in 1975.

The next time the Paleolithic diet gained an increase in popularity was during the 1990s. Ever since then, there is a growing amount of people using this way of nutrition, and they all have only good words for its effects. Various nutritional experts are now recommending this lifestyle if you want to achieve vitality and better health.

In fact, many other diets are nothing but variations of this diet. Mediterranean, Atkins, Soup diets all used the healthiest Paleo diet as a foundation. The results show that, if you want long-term success with your way of nutrition, Paleolithic lifestyle is still the best way to go.

The Science behind the Paleo Diet

Sure, you might like to know a thing or two from the Paleo diet history, but we all tend to put more belief in scientific research, So, let's take a look at what science thinks whether the Paleolithic way of nutrition is effective.

M. Konner and S. Boyd Eaton are among the leading researchers on the topic of the Paleo Diet. Their research was published in the New England Journal of Medicine with the following conclusions:

- The way how human genetic is constituted went through only small changes in the past 40,000 years
- Agriculture showed up 10,000 years ago but it only minimally affected our genes
- The Industrial Revolution and the implementation of modern techniques to process food happened too recently for it to have any effect on human evolution

- Therefore, nutritionists and physicians are inclined to believe that the factor behind the increased occurrence of hypertension, coronary heart diseases, certain cancer types, and diabetes is the habit of dieting implemented in the Western society

According to this research, modern diets are among the leading causes of the dominant health problems in the past 100 years or so. These aren't the only professionals that concluded this. Dr. Loren Cordain from the Colorado State University says the following:

"According to evidence gathered from DNA, the human genome changed very little in the last 40,000 years (less than 0.02%). Back then, our ancestors could find everything they needed in nature. That is why the experts believe that the human genome holds the secret to optimal nutrition that makes us healthy and fit."

Science also agrees that there are other significant benefits that Paleo diet has our health and well-being. In a research conducted by Ulrike Kmmerer and Rainer J Klement in 2011, the critical role of proper nutrition in preventing cancer was discovered.

The statistics are accurate – cancer is virtually unknown the primitive societies that focus or focused on hunting and gathering. That leads to a logical conclusion – the modern nutrition is the reason of this disease, especially grains and other carbohydrates. Thanks to their high content of gluten, lectins, and omega fatty acids, grains can lead to inflammation and cause various diseases. Restriction of carbs that is recommended by Paleo way of nutrition secures better control of blood sugar and improves cardiovascular health.

These are only several research studies that support the Paleo diet and its importance. The truth is that nutritional experts from around the world, as well as physicians and other doctors, agree that hunting-gathering way of nutrition should be the model how we should eat.

Why You Should Be on Paleo Diet

Most people choose the perfect way of nutrition for them based on the advantages that a particular diet brings. That being said, let's check out what are the health benefits of the Paleo diet and why it is your best choice. If you are among those who are keen on suspecting things, I included some scientific information to back up each of these Paleo benefits.

You Can Lose Weight

Science says: 66% of the adult Americans stated that they had issues with being overweight at least once in the last two years.

Although this might not be the most significant advantage, I believe it takes the top of the list for a considerable portion of the people reading this. It's true, one of the benefits of the Paleo diet is weight loss, but the emphasis should be on LONG-TERM weight loss.

You see, the Paleo way of nutrition won't just help you rich your ideal weight and shed those extra pounds. If you keep living the Paleolithic lifestyle, you will sustain that ideal weight for a long, long time. There are no side-effects or other reasons why you shouldn't use the Paleo diet for as long as you want, making it the ideal nutrition for everyone.

Your Cells Will Be Healthier

Science says: Cells are made from both saturated and unsaturated fats. Proper balance between the two is what secures their proper function.

Believe it or not, each cell in your organism is constituted from two types of fats, and your task is to ensure a healthy balance of the two. That way, you will make sure that the cells can send messages in and out and their job correctly. The Paleolithic nutrition guarantees healthy amounts of both saturated and unsaturated fats.

Your Brain Will Be Healthier

Science says: Omega-3 fatty acids play an integral role in proper functioning of the human brain, as well as its development and growth.

The average Western diet severely lacks in healthy Omega-3 fatty acids, which are crucial for our brain (and heart) health. Paleo diet recommends eating fatty fish, such as salmon and other cold water fish that contain a high amount of these acids.

Your Intestines Will Be Healthier

Science says: High amounts of refined carbs leads to spikes in blood sugar levels, which stimulates the creation of cytokines that are known to be inflammatory messengers.

Processed foods are the leading factor that causes inflammation within your GI tract. If you combine too much stress with too much junk food, you can even end up with the "leaky gut" syndrome, which leads to your intestinal walls being breached.

If you start the Paleo nutrition and keep that lifestyle, you will secure that your gastrointestinal tract remains healthy. On top of that, you will ensure better digestion and proper absorption of all the nutrients from healthy foods you consume.

You Can Boost Your Immune System

Science says: Various studies relate Omega-3 fatty acids with reduced inflammation throughout the body. It is considered that they can help in fighting cancer, heart disease, and arthritis.

Inflammation is the primary cause of cardiovascular health issues. Considering that the Paleo diet is based on sound nutritional principles, it contains a bunch of anti-inflammatory foods that can significantly reduce the risk of inflammation and boost your immune system.

You Will Feel More Energized

Science says: The sugars from foods that have a low glycemic index are absorbed slowly. That helps people overcome the lack of energy felt after eating a high amount of refined carbs or sugars.

The popularity of energy drinks became so apparent during the last decade or two. The reason why people have been feeling the lack of energy is not stress, but the nutrition that plainly sucks! Just take a look at it this way – your breakfast is usually a bagel full of cheese accompanies by a cup of coffee filled with sugar. That is the best way to get yourself ridden of the energy you need for the day. Unlike that, the Paleo diet promotes eating foods that provide more energy for your body.

Improved Tolerance to Glucose and Help in Fighting Diabetes

Science says: 1.4 million Americans are diagnosed with type 2 diabetes each year.

You might think that it's still not that part of life when you should worry about diabetes. In fact, now is the perfect time because you can maybe prevent diabetes in the future by improving the insulin resistance now. The Paleo diet is an excellent way to improve the glucose metabolism of your body.

If you already have diabetes, the Paleo lifestyle is also the right choice in that case. Not only Paleolithic diet improves your insulin resistance, but it also helps prevent blood sugar spikes in the human body. That means that you can quickly put your diabetes under control. In some cases, you might not even need the medications to live with it.

Is this not enough for you? Let's take a look at some other benefits of the Paleo diet:

- It reduces bloat – if you want a flatter stomach, you should consider reducing bloat. You can that by increasing your fiber intake and drinking more water, which are both in line with the Paleo nutrition
- It's filling – even though you will probably eat less when on the Paleo diet, you will feel more satiated. The reason for that are the nutrients that are filling. Eating less and feeling satiety will help you reach and maintain your ideal weight
- Better sleep – if you have been feeling sleep-deprived, Paleo diet can help you get regular night sleep back

Complete Food Guide
for Paleo Diet

If you are new to the Paleo diet or you worry that it's overly restrictive, I hope that our food guide will resolve all dilemmas when it comes to what you can eat while on this way of nutrition. Before we dive in into particular categories, let's take a look at a short list of things that you can consume:

- Vegetables
- Fruits
- Meat
- Seafood
- Nuts and seeds
- Unrefined oils

As you can see, there are plenty of choices to make within the allowed types of foods. We will later talk about things that you need to avoid, but let's now dive in into particular categories of foods that you can eat.

Foods to Eat

- **Meat**

Proteins are an integral part of the Paleo nutrition and protein that we get from animal sources are one of the healthiest ones you can find. Believe it or not, meat is considered to be one of the foundations of a Paleo diet. Of course, you should always bear in mind that you should consume natural meat. That means that you should avoid processed versions of it, such as ham, bacon or hot dogs.

The other condition that you should fulfill is that you should look for wild and grass-fed meat whenever that is an option (as often as possible). Aside from that, you are absolutely free to choose the types of meat you want to eat. You can be adventurous when it comes to the ways to prepare the meat (baking, steaming) and choose different cuts.

You can consume red meat, including lamb, beef, veal, goat, buffalo, venison, elk, and bison. As for poultry, you also have a broad range at your disposal, such as turkey, chicken, duck, pheasant, geese, partridge, emu, quail, ostrich, and so on. You don't have to stop there if you have the chance, feel free to try rabbit, moose, wild boar, reindeer, alligator, or even turtle.

- **Seafood**

Seafood is considered as the other staple of the Paleo diet. Just like land animals, the one you find in the sea are an incredible source of healthy nutrients and protein. They secure us the required dose of Omega-3 fatty acids, which is crucial for our heart health, as well as other important vitamins and nutrients. If it's possible, you should look for wild-caught fish and avoid those who have been exposed to the toxins found in the environment.

The list of fish that you can consume is long, and we didn't order it by its health benefits, so you can feel free to choose any from this list: anchovy, mackerel, catfish, cuttlefish, swai, bass, cod, prawns, flounder, sole, oysters, shark, crab, lobster, clams, walleye, sardines, herring, squid, perch, bluefish, crayfish, octopus, tuna, barracuda, scallops, trout, snapper, salmon, halibut, swordfish, mussels...

- **Vegetables**

Our parents were talking to us that vegetables are healthy and they did it for a reason. Most of the vegetables are incredibly rich in fiber, as well as other integral nutrients, such as minerals and vitamins. That is why their inclusion into the Paleo diet is an absolute must. Of course, you should look to choose different veggies whenever you have the chance because they are not all equal when it comes to their nutritional value. However, you have so many vegetables to choose from that I'm sure you will find loads of them you love to consume.

- o **Cruciferous vegetables:** broccoli, Brussels sprouts, cauliflower, horseradish, daikon, radish, kohlrabi, rutabaga
- o **Leafy greens:** spinach, kale, beet greens, turnip greens, cabbage, collard greens, watercress, mustard greens, Swiss chard, radicchio, bok choy, arugula, lettuce
- o **Safe starchy veggies** (moderate consummation): sweet potatoes, carrots, cassava, taro, parsnips, yams

o **Squashes:** spaghetti squash, butternut, yellow squash, zucchini, acorn, pumpkin, Kabocha squash, Mexican gray squash
o **Other vegetables:** Seaweed, jicama, beets, cucumbers, cactus, shallots, green onions, leeks, fennel, garlic, celery, onion, artichoke, sweet peppers, hot peppers, bell peppers, eggplant, asparagus

As you can see, there are plenty of veggies at your disposal on the Paleo diet, so feel free to mix and match any way you like.

- **Fruits**

Fruits are rich in fructose, which is a type of sugar. However, considering that it is nature's sugar, the Paleo experts recommend consuming fruits in moderation. After all, they are certainly a much better option than refined sugars and packaged candies. You should always look to consume fruit in its natural form, although you can allow yourself a smoothie here and there. Two things to avoid are artificial fruit juices and packaged fruit, which usually contain added sugar.

The experts don't recommend going over three servings of fruit every day.

- o **Berries:** raspberries, cranberries, blackberries, blueberries, strawberries, currants, goji berries, bilberries, elderberries, acai
  - o **Citrus:** tangerines, lemons, limes, pomelos, grapefruits, oranges
  - o **Stone fruit:** apricots, nectarines, peaches
  - o **Other:** pineapple, tomatoes, mango, bananas, papaya, watermelon, avocado, apples, coconuts, guava, figs, cantaloupe, tomatillos, grapes, honeydew, plantains

- **Nuts and Seeds**

Considering that the Paleo diet excludes grains (we'll get to that later), there are other viable alternatives when it comes to baked goods. For example, you can use coconut or almond flour to make bread, cakes, pies, and even cereals. If you are a fan of milk, you can always choose coconut or almond options, as well as nut butter, which are also appropriate for the Paleo lifestyle. However, you should consume nuts in moderation, considering that they are rich in calories.

- o **Nuts:** almonds, hazelnuts, walnuts, Macadamia nuts, pine nuts, pecans,
  - o **Seeds:** sunflower seeds, pumpkin seeds, flax seeds, sesame seeds

- **Friendly fats**

Although fat has been demonized by the media in the past couple of decades, the truth is that there are friendly fats that are extremely healthy and our organism needs them. That being said, you should avoid using any refined and processed options and concentrate on natural alternatives, which offer improved nutritional value. You can also find some healthy fats in certain oils.

- o **Fats:** tallow, lard, ghee, rendered animal fats
- o **Oils:** olive oil, avocado oil, flaxseed oil, coconut oil, walnut oil

Now that we've seen what foods you are allowed to eat let's take a look at foods that you should avoid.

Foods to Avoid

The list of foods that you cannot eat on a Paleo diet is actually the list of foods that can create chaos in your organism. Not only they negatively affect your health, but they can also be an obstacle to your goal to reaching your ideal weight. Here is the food that you should avoid when living a Paleo lifestyle:

- **Grains**

Even though the American official Food Guide Pyramid recommends grains and even though you might have eaten them since you were a kid, the first thing to cut out when on Paleo diet are grains. Giving up wheat means that you will cut out bread or bagels, which might not be easy, but it will have an incredibly positive effect.

We mentioned already that grains have toxic anti-nutrients, which irritate our gastrointestinal tract and cause the damage to gut lining. Aside from that, they are one of the primary causes of fat storage in your body because they cause the release of insulin when consumed. Even after a couple of days without grains, you should feel more energized, and your digesting should be better.

To avoid: Wheat, oats, corn, rye, spelt, quinoa, rice, buckwheat, barley, amaranth, millet...

- **Fast Food**

When you think about it, our ancestors didn't have the opportunity to visit fast food restaurants, which is why we should steer clear of them, too. There is not a single thing you can purchase in this type of restaurants that are considered fitting with the Paleo diet. If you don't trust me, take a look at the Super Size Me documentary.

To avoid: Burgers, French fries, everything else from fast food restaurants

- **Added Sugar**

While you can't eliminate sugar completely from your diet (fructose or fruit sugar is still sugar), you should focus on avoiding added or refined types. Not only they cause spikes in blood sugar levels, which can create chaos in your body, but they also diminish your weight loss efforts.

To avoid: White sugar, brown sugar, corn syrup, rice syrup, molasses, packaged sugar, stevia, agave, aspartame...

- **Processed Foods**

Processed foods, by rule, contain artificial ingredients, such as artificial coloring and a bunch of chemicals and additives. That is why, when you visit the store, if you notice that food is packed in a colorful box, the chances are that you should avoid it.

To avoid: All food with artificial ingredients, such as coloring, additives or other chemicals

- **Seed and Industrial Oils**

Our ancestors didn't figure out the technique how to make their oil last for months. However, the food producers today add artificial ingredients and unhealthy trans fats to secure that their oil will last longer. That, in turn, makes those oils unhealthy, which means that you should steer clear of them.

To avoid: Canola oil, sunflower oil, cottonseed oil, safflower oil, peanut oil, corn oil, palm kernel oil, margarine...

- **Legumes**

This one might surprise you because legumes technically do come from the earth. However, they contain phytic acid, which is considered an anti-nutrient (it's the same toxic ingredient that you can find in grains). Unfortunately, there is no use in soaking or sprouting them either because they are rich in carbs which make them harder for digestion.

To avoid: Peas, black beans, white beans, broad beans, chickpeas, lentils, soybeans, peanuts...

- **White Potatoes**

Another food that can be found on the ground but you should avoid it. In the ancient times, potatoes were not that easy to grow, which is why our ancestors probably discovered them a bit later when our biological designed wasn't prepared to digest them properly.

White potatoes are high in starch and sugar content, and they stimulate the release of insulin. Aside from that, they can be the factor of intestinal distress. You should be especially careful when they start turning green. That means that chaconine and solanine appeared; those are substances toxic to insects and predators but also to humans.

- **Dairy**

Believe it or not, we are the only species on Earth that consume milk that was given by another animal. Aside from that, we are the only ones who believe that we need milk after we pass the weaning period. Unlike the popular belief that it's healthy, cow's milk should serve to help calves grow quickly. Aside from that, when this milk is processed, we also find additional probiotics, bacteria, hormones, and even antibiotics. I wouldn't say that's a real or natural food, which is why you should steer clear of it.

By rule, you should avoid all dairy, but there is one type that can be included -

To avoid: Milk, yogurt, half-and-half, sour cream, cheese

- **Sodas**

Although they technically fall into the category of both foods that are processed and that have added sugar, we are putting special emphasis on sodas just to be clear how bad they are. The nutritional value of your average soda is close to none. They are empty carbs full of artificial ingredients and are among the causes of many diseases, including heart disease, high blood pressure, diabetes, obesity, and cancer. As soon as you manage to exclude them, you will notice feeling much better in only a day or two.

Dining Out Guide

Sticking to the Paleo nutrition when you dine out is hard, especially if your friends are not on the same nutrition as you. Before you even head out for dinner with them, you should explain that you made a lifestyle change and that you expect, at the least, their support. That should mean that they should avoid teasing you or making jokes. It also means that they would agree to go to a Paleo friendly restaurant so that you can have a proper meal that fits with your plan of nutrition.

Knowing which restaurant you will go to is the first step to take if you plan on dining out. Preparation is essential because you don't want to end up in some junk food restaurant where you can't even have the option of eating a healthy meal. Do your research and check the area as I'm sure you can find a Paleo-friendly restaurant. Once you do, ask your friends to go out there. If you ask me, Mexican restaurants can be a good choice, but you can also go with sushi or seafood.

Once you arrive at the restaurant, you need to avoid the urge to stuff your face with appetizers. Be strong, order the main course and patiently wait for it. Maybe you can ask the waiter to skip bringing appetizers, but that may not be polite to your friends. But, even if you see them on the table, you can always skip eating them. Instead, you can spend the time waiting for the main dish talking to your friends. If you absolutely need to have something, make sure to ask the waiter to bring you a side salad while you are waiting for the entrée.

When choosing your main course, you should be careful with the sides. Most restaurants offer multiple choices when it comes to sides, which is why you should take a look at them and select the option that is most Paleo-friendly. For example, if French fries are an option for the sides, you can probably ask to bring Sweet potato fries as an alternative. They will be equally delicious, but far healthier.

You should also be careful when it comes to dressings. A bit of olive oil won't harm, but most of the dressings today contain artificial and processed ingredients. Make sure to ask your waiter on how the restaurant prepares the dressing and, if it didn't sound right, ask him to bring it separately or don't bring it at all.

In general, you shouldn't be wary of speaking to the staff of the restaurant, especially the waiter. He's there to be at your service, and it's in his interest for you to be satisfied. If he does everything right and tries hard to fulfill your requests, don't forget to be generous with your tip.

According to people I have been talking to, dessert is the time when most of us can't prone the temptation of failing the Paleo way of nutrition. That is why you should make sure to skip it and get some tea or coffee instead. That way, you not only benefit from the positive effects of those drinks, but you also avoid additional carbs and sugar that are usually in desserts.

While we are on the subjects of drinks, if you are out celebrating with your friends, you should know that the Paleo diet doesn't support alcohol. You can always offer to be the driver to avoid anyone offering it during the evening.

Nutritional Supplements

The Paleo diet is one of the most nutrient-dense ways of nutrition out there. That being said, it's not that common for a nutrient deficiency to appear when living Paleo lifestyle. On the other hand, most people are eating a modern Paleo diet, and most of us adapt the way of nutrition to ourselves and the food we like. So, for example, we end up not taking the leanest and the healthiest piece of meat.

Let's take a look at some of the reasons when a nutritional deficiency may appear:

- Disease
- Pregnancy
- Old age (not always)
- A highly restrictive diet
- Unusual weather conditions (no sun for a long time)

The Paleo way of nutrition fits into the restrictive diet so, depending on an individual and their choice, it might cause a nutritional deficiency in some cases (for example, if you are going pegan). I know, you are going to tell me that our ancestor certainly didn't take supplements. That's true, but they also ate exclusively grass-fed meat and wild-caught fish. And is that something that you can claim for yourself today? Aside from that, the pollution of air is far worse today, and you probably have a history with junk food that our ancestors didn't have.

It might be best to consult with your doctor before choosing whether you need supplements. Here are some that are mostly used by people on Paleo diet:

Vitamin D

We get this vitamin from sunlight and food (mostly fish). However, the sun plays a larger role in securing us the vitamin D that we need for our body to work properly. In cases when sun exposure is low, making it up with food is a tricky task. A recent survey showed that about 40% of Americans lack enough vitamin D and that is something that cannot be changed even with perfect nutrition.

Vitamin D has a bunch of positive effects on our health, including that it's important for our heart and brain, which is why you might consider a vitamin D supplement if you don't get much sun.

Fish oil

It's always a better option to eat actual fish to get your healthy Omega-3 fatty acids. However, if you are not a fan of fish, you can get some benefits from fish oil supplements. Fish oil positively affects your heart health and has an anti-inflammatory effect.

There is one thing to keep in mind – if your nutrition is filled with unhealthy fats, fish oil can't magically erase them. Fortunately, if you follow the Paleo diet, you will prevent the intake of unhealthy fats.

Magnesium

Have you been experiencing muscle cramps? Are you under a lot of stress lately? Magnesium can help you in these situations. Aside from that, it is known as a mild laxative, so you might consider it for dealing with constipation issues, too.

These are some general supplement suggestions for Paleo diet. If you fall into one of the risk categories when it comes to nutritional deficiencies (you are pregnant or have a disease at the moment), you might need additional supplements. The best idea is to consult your doctor before starting Paleo diet.

Starting the Paleo Diet

Regardless of the name of the diet you chose, they all share one similarity; they are extremely tricky to stick to during the beginning phase. The reason behind this is simple; starting a diet means that you need to change your lifestyle and make a bunch of changes to your everyday habits at once. That is not an easy job, so let's take a look at some advice that might help you.

Adjusting Your Mindset

There is one thing that you need to clear up in your mind before you begin the Paleo lifestyle. Your primary goal might be to shed those extra pounds, but that might be the wrong approach. While you can use it for motivation, your ultimate objective should be to change your relationship toward food and how you see it. Your goal should be to get used to nutrition that benefits your overall health and a lifestyle you can live with permanently. Just remember, you are in it for yourself; think about the health issues and the extra pounds you have and reflect on how Paleo diet can assist you in improving your overall health and well-being. That should be motivating enough to start.

When starting the Paleo diet, it doesn't come as strange that you think that it is overly restrictive. You might be in just a day or two, but you already start feeling like it's limiting you too hard. It might be because you just decided to completely give up the food you enjoyed until a couple of days ago, and you gave it up FOREVER. That last word sticks in your mind and subconscious starts playing games with you, making you desire processed foods or candies even more.

There is a neat trick you can apply to slowly adjust your mindset and get accustomed to your diet. Promise yourself that you will follow the Paleo way of nutrition for two or three weeks just to see its effects. If so many people succeeded, why not give it a shot? Before you start, use your phone or a camera to take a picture of yourself. Also, stand on the scale and write down your weight.

During the trial period, make sure to follow all the Paleo diet guidelines. Throw out dairy and grains from your nutrition, start consuming fruits and veggies, focus on meat and avoid sugar and liquid calories. Once the trial period is done, stand in front of the mirror and compare yourself to the image you've made before you started. Also, ask yourself – are you feeling better? If you followed the Paleo principles, I'm sure the answer will be yes.

Aside from making sure that the diet works, your new look (and feel) should give you the motivation to continue with the Paleo diet. Furthermore, you will find that you don't miss that junk food anymore. Instead, you feel much happier to have a fresh piece of fruit. That will be the first sign that you have won the battle for a healthier lifestyle within your mind.

How to Make a Successful Transition to Paleo Lifestyle

The first thing to remember is the mistake most people are making - they jump in too quickly. Changing your way of nutrition is a change of lifestyle, and that causes some severe adjustments. That is why you shouldn't be too strict in the beginning. In fact, if you don't want to make the trial period approach I suggested in the previous section, you can transit to Paleo lifestyle gradually. If you decide to go that way, you should know that you won't maximize the positive effects of the Paleo diet at once. Regardless of that, the slower transition might be a better fit for you, and it's a legit approach.

There are two different methods you can try:

- Phasing out one group at a time – in this case, you will throw out each food group from your nutrition one by one. You should start with sugar and continue with dairy products, wheat, and finally legumes and beans
- Phasing out one meal at a time – when using this approach, you should start by making all your snacks completely paleo. The next move is to ensure that your dinners are Paleolithic, lunch and finally breakfast. You can also start by making one meal everyday Paleo the first week and then increase it to two, three, etc. every next week.

Here are some other tips you can try when starting the Paleo diet

Clean up your kitchen

There is a good chance that your kitchen is full of grains, candies, and other unhealthy foods at this point. The first thing you need to do is get a garbage bag and throw out all the things that don't fit with the Paleo nutrition. If you don't want to waste food, you can always pack it up and give it away to the local object serving those in need.

Plan your meals in advance

Another sound advice regardless of what type of nutrition you choose is to make a plan of your meals at least two or three days in advance. You should always know what you are going to eat and you should make sure that your fridge is full of food that fits with the Paleo lifestyle. You should also adjust the shopping lists accordingly to make it easier to stick to your new diet.

Share your idea with others

Don't be afraid to share with the world that you've switched to Paleo nutrition. Furthermore, you should ask the ones that are living with you (family, partner) to join you because Paleo lifestyle is incredibly healthy for anyone. If they say no, then the least they could do is to offer support and encourage you on your new path. You should make them promise you that they wouldn't try to entice you with unhealthy food while you are working to adjust to Paleo lifestyle.

Don't dwell on mistakes

It's only normal to suffer a setback every once in a while. It can happen for different reasons; you might feel down because of the high amount of stress at work, or you just weren't able to resist the temptation while celebrating with friends. You've eaten some processed foods or sweets, so what? It's not the end of the world. The important thing now is not to dwell on your mistakes and hop back on the wagon with your next meal.

Don't be easygoing

Although you shouldn't dwell on mistakes, you should know that each change to the style of nutrition requires some degree of sacrifice. That means that you should be prepared to fight your cravings and urges because that is the only way to achieve your objectives and become a healthier and better-looking person. You should find the right balance; there is no need for your diet to be too hard for you, but you should be ready to go through a little trouble for a good cause.

Remember what your motivation is

Do you want to extend your lifespan so that you can see your grandson head for college? Would you like to solve your issues with obesity and become agiler? Are you just looking to transform your body to look better for the next summer? Whatever your motivation, make sure to remind yourself of it and hang in there.

Don't forget to stay hydrated

Hydration is important on Paleo diet, especially during the beginning phase when you might face increased urination. That is why you want to make sure that you compensate by drinking enough water.

Salt is your friend

Changing to a low-carb diet usually means that you release a significant amount of sodium through urination. However, sodium is an essential electrolyte, especially for your kidneys, and you need to make sure that you compensate for this loss. Lack of sodium can be the factor of some side effects when you start the Paleo diet. That is why you should consume enough salt, which is the best source of sodium. You should use broth or bouillon, or you can even drink a cup of salted water.

Is Paleo an Expensive Diet?

After taking a look at what living the Paleo lifestyle means, most people start thinking that it is an expensive way of life. Although there are cheaper diets out there, Paleo nutrition is the healthiest options you can choose for your body. There are some tips that you can use to make Paleo more fitting with your budget.

How to Eat Paleo on a Budget

It's not true that a Paleo diet can be expensive. As long as you follow these tips, you can make the Paleo nutrition more affordable.

Set Priorities Straight

I'm sure that you are spending loads of money on things you don't even need during the month. How can you say then that there is not enough space in your budget for a healthy diet? On average, Paleo nutrition increases monthly food budget for about $100. While that may seem like a lot, I'm sure that you can make a couple of cuts here and there and make sure that you don't feel that additional amount you spend on groceries.

Try to change your priorities to what's expensive. After all, you can't put a price on your health, but you definitely can afford to miss the latest episode of the show on that pay-per-view channel.

Spend Less Time Shopping

This advice is also significant because it will help you avoid all those unhealthy foods easier. You see, most supermarkets and other grocery stores are built the same way – processed food is located in the middle while fruits, veggies, and meat are allocated on the edges of the store. That is why you should apply the technique of buying in a circle. You shouldn't even go to the center of the supermarket, keep to the edges and proceed to checkout as soon as you get everything from your list. That way you will ensure that you don't buy something you might not need and save some money.

Shop at a Local Farmer's Market

An even better alternative to a grocery store is to visit your local farmer's market. Believe it or not, virtually everything in there is Paleo-friendly. Aside from that, you might find that the food is more affordable, absolutely fresh and maybe even more delicious than the one from the supermarket.

Look for Discounts

When you truly need to save some money, you can always search for discounts in the supermarket. For example, grocery stores often discount the meat that is close to its "sell by" date. There is nothing to worry about – the meat is still good! However, make sure to cook it as soon as possible so that the "sell by" date doesn't expire while the meat is in your fridge.

Stay at Home

The best way to make sure that you will save some money is to avoid eating out. That might be tricky because you want to hang out with your friends or have a fancy dinner with your partner, but staying at home and preparing own meals will save some money.

Buy in Bulk

If you don't mind eating the same type of meat for several days, you can also buy in bulk. For example, you can purchase a bag of chicken thighs and save some money compared to purchasing only what you need for a single meal. You can also use some of the online delivery systems. Just make sure to freeze the food that you are not consuming right away and thaw it once you plan to eat it.

As already mentioned, it's all about changing your perspective. Paleo diet can bring incredible benefits to your health and overall well-being, and that is something that's worth spending couple more bucks.

Risks and Concerns

Just like any restricting diet, the Paleo way of nutrition also comes with its portions of risks and concerns. Fortunately, there are not many side effects because this is one of the healthiest diets out there, but let's take a look at some things that you need to be aware of when making a transition to the Paleo lifestyle. The important thing to know is that you

Low-Carb Flu

The Paleo diet's primary requirement is to reduce your carb intake. Considering that most people were on the modern diet before making the change, the transition often means that their intake of carbs is dramatically reduced. However, our bodies are designed with metabolic flexibility, which means that they have the ability to change between using carbohydrates and fat for energy. Up until now, you've probably been consuming a mixture of carbs and fats, and you felt okay. But, the excessive amount of carbs led to weight issues and maybe even health problems.

Now that you've decided to make a change to the low-carb diet, such as Paleo, your body should adjust to using only fat as fuel. While our organisms are designed to do that, it takes a couple of days (no more than a week if you stick to the rules of Paleo) to adjust. During those days you might experience so-called low-carb flu.

The symptoms of low-carb flu are:

- **Fogginess or fuzziness** – you feel like your brain is just not working properly. Can come combined with headaches
- **Crankiness** – you might feel irritated for no apparent reason
- **Lack of energy** – exercising seems like a challenge you just can't complete. You feel very exhausted
- **Craving for carbs** – you feel incredible hunger and the desire to eat everything in sight, especially, pizza, pasta, or candy

If you experience some of these symptoms, you don't have to worry. You are not sick, but your body is adapting to your new way of nutrition. The good news is that the low-carb flu usually lasts for only two or three days. It usually occurs between days 2 and 7 of your Paleo nutrition, and it doesn't happen to everyone; some people don't experience any of the symptoms.

And the best part is that, once you go through that initial phase, you will turn your body into a fat-burning machine. You will feel happier and more energized than ever, and you will start noticing the effects on your weight. This side effect might be a problem in the short term, but it is worth the pain because there is a long term gain.

The best way to try to avoid the low-carb flu is to make sure that you consume enough water and to secure the intake of electrolytes. In case you feel like you have some of the symptoms, you might make it better by drinking a glass of salted water to get some sodium into your organism. Just make sure that you are using healthy salt option, such as Himalayan salt.

Other Side Effects

While low-carb flu is the side effect that is hardest to avoid, here are some other things that can happen during the initial phase of the Paleo diet.

Ketogenic Breath

As your body is going through the change from using carbs to using fat as energy, you will enter a process known as ketosis. During that period, you will get rid of the toxins in your organism. Among other ways, you will do so by respiration. One of the toxins found in human body is acetone, which you will also expel by breathing. As you might know, because it is used for removing nail polish, acetone has a distinct scent, which some people might not like. The breath that smells of acetone is known as ketogenic breath, and it can show up during the initial phase of the Paleo diet. There's nothing to worry about, simply take a mint and be patient until you expel all the excess acetone from your body,w which shouldn't last more than two weeks.

Hypothyroidism

This issue occurs only when you go too far with your Paleo diet. The task of the Paleolithic nutrition is to suppress your appetite. As a result, your body might enter a so-called starvation mode. At that moment, it will downregulate the function of your thyroid to save some energy. That is something that happens if you lose too much weight, especially in a short period. That is why you should not look to be too thin, at least now immediately.

The symptoms of hypothyroidism include sluggishness, fatigue, and sensitivity to cold. The best way to avoid this is to increase the amount of vegetables you consume and keep it at a high level.

Cravings

It's only natural that you feel cravings for the food you consumed up until a couple of days ago. Don't be surprised if you have incredible cravings for potato chips or candies, especially during the initial phase of Paleo diet. However, once you push through this starting period, you will find yourself no longer wanting any sweets or treats because you will develop a habit of living without them.

Constipation

Your digestive system also needs some time to adapt to all the changes coming with the Paleo diet, which is exactly why constipation might occur in some cases. However, you should avoid it simply by making sure that you drink enough water and securing enough electrolytes. Foods rich in fiber are also an excellent choice.

Physical Performance

In the beginning phase, Paleo diet might influence your physical performance. However, be aware that this is only for a short period and you can go back to exercising to your maximum in a week or two. Furthermore, you will feel extra energized once your body starts using only fat as fuel. There is an incredible number of famous athletes on the Paleo diet, and they all achieve better results than their competition.

Conclusion

Thank you again for purchasing this book!

I hope this book was able to help you understand the Paleo diet and all it benefits properly.

As you could see, Paleo has an enormous number of health and other benefits. This book had the goal of giving you an in-depth look at this healthy way of nutrition and how it works. Aside from that, you now know which foods you can eat and which you should avoid, as well as all other information relevant for this diet.

The only thing you should remember on your path to weight loss with a Paleo diet is to stay strong. I know that it's not easy to fight cravings, but the results will be more than worth it. Putting in just a small effort can get you a long way.

Finally, if you enjoyed this book, then I'd like to ask you for a favor, would you be kind enough to leave a review for this book on Amazon? It'd be greatly appreciated.

Visit the link below to leave a review:
https://www.amazon.com/review/create-review
For more information, please check out my blog at:
Mastering-life.com

Thank you and good luck!

Preview of

"Ketogenic Diet" Book

Introduction

I want to thank you and congratulate you for downloading the book "**Ketogenic Diet**"

This book contains proven steps and strategies on how to lose weight with the ketogenic diet.

I used to have a big problem with obesity. I was constantly eating and overeating unhealthy and junk food and I didn't lift a finger when it comes to activity. One day I've decided – things have got to change!

The ketogenic diet helped me not only achieve my ideal weight (I lost over 50 pounds), but it also improved my body composition by getting rid of that stored fat in my belly and other areas.

Now, I look and feel much better! I have so much energy and I can go on and on without feeling tired. That is why I've decided to share with you the secret of achieving the perfect state of your organism with the help of the ketogenic diet.

Here's what we will cover in this book:

- What is ketogenic diet, how it works and why it is a perfectly healthy way to lose weight

- How to calculate the number of macronutrients you need?

- What food should you eat and avoid during keto?

- 4-week ketogenic diet plan as a suggestion

- More than 30 completely keto-friendly recipes!

And much more!

I've used my own experience of going through keto to help explain it to you in the best way. I noted down all the questions I had and tried to answer them for you in this book.

Everything you need to know about the ketogenic diet is in one place – here.

Thanks again for downloading this book, I hope you enjoy it!

Chapter 1 – Ketosis Explained

Ketosis is a regular metabolic process in our body and it happens on an everyday basis. It is a metabolic state where your body uses ketone bodies in the blood for some of its energy supply.

The human body is extremely adjustable and it can process different nutrients into the fuel it needs to work. Carbs, fats, and proteins are all potential sources of energy supply. When you eat a lot of carbohydrates or proteins, your body breaks them down into glucose (also known as blood sugar). Glucose is then used in creating an energy molecule called ATP, which your organism uses for maintenance and daily activities within the body.

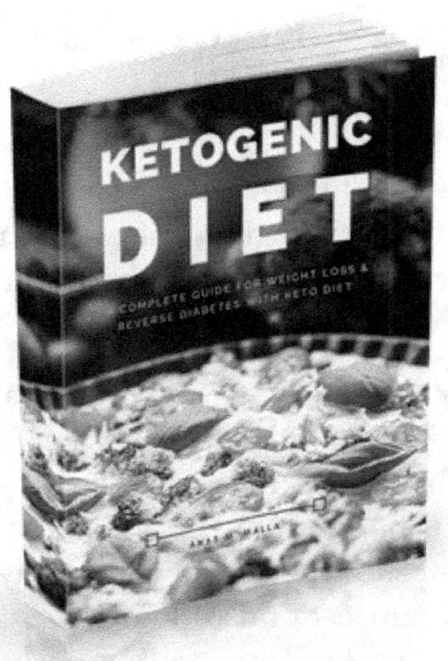

Believe it or not, our body uses most of the nutrients we intake just for daily maintenance. However, if you eat enough food, the chances are that there will be an excessive amount of glucose which the body doesn't require at the moment. In that case, one of the two things happens:

- **Glycogenesis** – the excess amount of glucose is converted to glycogen and stored in your muscles and liver

- **Lipogenesis** – once your body believes that there is enough glycogen in your liver and muscles, the remaining glucose will be converted into fats and stored within your body

Ketosis is a process that happens when your organism is out of glycogen or glucose. In cases when your body can't access food, it will start burning fat and creating ketones (energy molecules). This process usually occurs when you are sleeping, so it is a completely normal metabolic state of the organism. The human body has a natural ability to switch metabolic pathways.

When your body starts burning fat and making fatty acids, the end result of the process is the creation of ketones. These molecules are then used by your brain and muscles as a fuel. In most cases, the human body uses glucose as the main source of its energy supply. However, once the carbohydrate or protein intake is low, your body will simply use fatty acids as a natural alternative.

What Is Ketosis and How Does It Work?

Ketosis is a process that occurs when your body is out of glycogen or glucose and it starts using consumed and stored fat as a fuel for maintenance and daily activities. It is a metabolic state your body should be in when you are on a ketogenic diet.

The study conducted by the University of California shows that the human organism actually prefers using ketones. In fact, it is about 70% more efficient than when running on glucose. If you think about it from an evolutionary point of view, it makes perfect sense. Our ancestors didn't have constant access to glucose. Hell, they didn't even have regular access to food.

Instead, their body was using the fat from the animal they ate.

The Process Explained

Your liver breaks down the consumed or stored fat and releases fatty acid molecules and glycerol. The next step is breaking down the fatty acids further. This process is called ketogenesis and it produces a ketone body by the name of acetoacetate.

Your body converts acetoacetate into one of the two types of ketones:

- **BHB (beta-hydroxybutyrate)** – after your body gets adapted to the state of ketosis, your muscles will use the acetoacetate to convert it to BHB and your body will then use it as brain fuel

- **Acetone** – lesser amounts of acetone are converted into glucose, but most of it is thrown out as waste. This might lead to a characteristic breath smell that ketogenic dieters are familiar with

As your organism gets used to ketosis, your body will expel a lesser amount of ketones. This doesn't mean that the process is slowing down. It just means that your body got better at feeding the brain with BHB as an energy supply.

You do need glucose in small amounts to maintain good health, which is why your organism creates it with acetone. The liver is there to make sure that you have enough glucose in your blood.

Unlike glucose, there is absolutely no need for carbohydrates. More than 50% of the excessive amount of proteins is turned into glucose. That is why eating carbs is a bad thing if you are on a ketogenic diet – it can knock you out of the state of ketosis.

Ketosis vs. Starvation

The state of ketosis is not the same as fasting. Starvation occurs when you don't have any food source whatsoever. It leads to your body using your muscle tissues to make the glucose it needs.

On the other hand, ketosis is a healthy way to lose additional pounds. The ketogenic process helps your body use the amount of fat it has stored and helps you preserve your muscle tissue.

Go to this link to check out the rest of the "**Ketogenic Diet**":

http://amzn.to/2ps3ePm

Check Out My Other Books

Below you'll find some of my other popular books that are popular on Amazon and Kindle as well. Simply click on the links below to check them out.

Alternatively, you can visit my "Author Page" on Amazon to see other work done by me:

Anas Malla: http://amzn.to/2nzCevB

- **Alkaline Diet V.1**
  http://amzn.to/2shityl

- **Ketogenic Diet**
  http://amzn.to/2ps3ePm

- **Ketogenic Bread Cookbook V.1**
  http://amzn.to/2m8hixm

- **Ketogenic Bread Cookbook V.2**
  http://amzn.to/2r3qsPJ

- **Ketogenic Bread Cookbook V.3**
  http://amzn.to/2r3Af8j

- **Instant Pot Ketogenic Cookbook V.1**
  http://amzn.to/2o4oCfP

- **Instant Pot Ketogenic Cookbook V.2**
  http://amzn.to/2o4oCfP

- **Ketogenic Fat Bombs V.1**
  http://amzn.to/2qDgS4U

- **Minimalist Living**
  http://amzn.to/2phTu8M

- **Conversation Tactics**
  http://amzn.to/2oj23Qg

If the links do not work, for whatever reason, you can simply search for these titles on the Amazon website to find them.